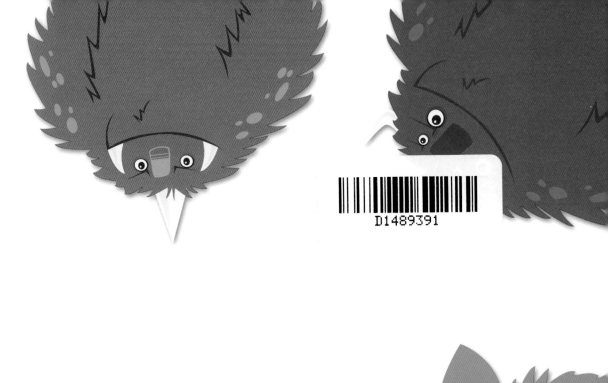

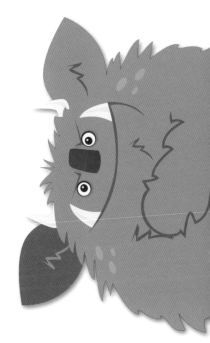

Compliments of
Stony Brook
MS Comprehensive
Care Center

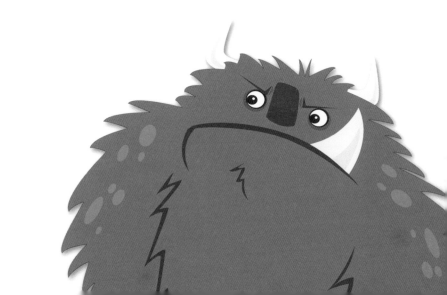

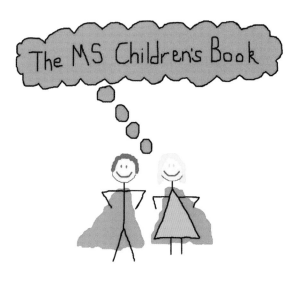

The MS Children's Book

Special thanks to Kenneth Yuen.

MS Children's Book

Copyright © 2011 by Zac Raasch

Requests for permission to make copies of any part of the work should be submitted online at info@mascotbooks.com or mailed to Mascot Books, 560 Herndon Parkway #120, Herndon, VA 20170

PRT0611A

Printed in the United States.

ISBN-13: 978-1-936319-63-3
ISBN-10: 1-936319-63-2

www.mascotbooks.com

MS CHILDREN'S BOOK

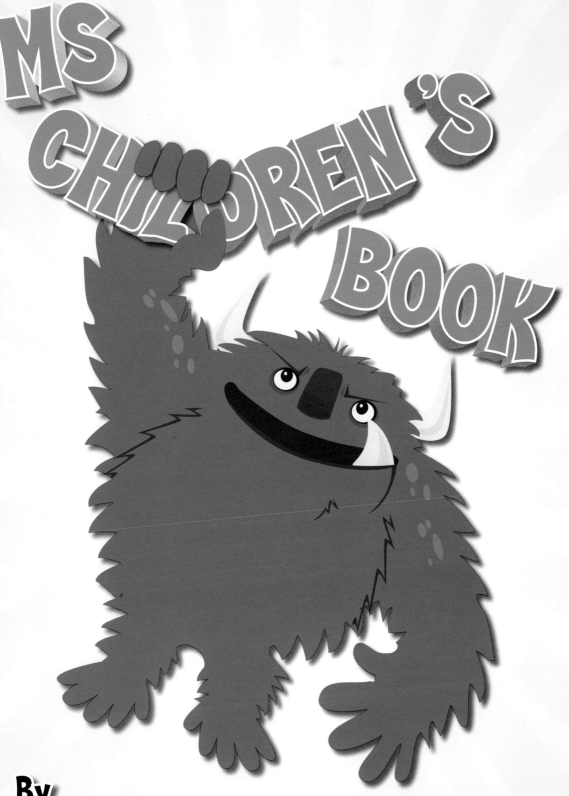

By
Zac Raasch

illustrated by
Amy Donohoe

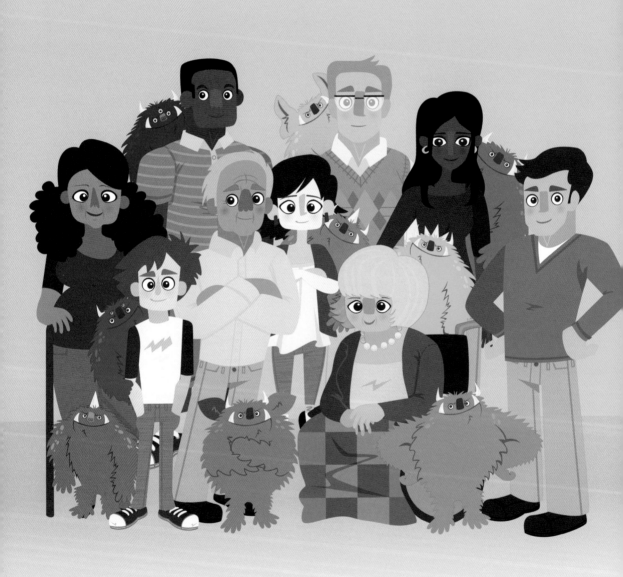

This here is My Sick–
Multiple Sclerosis.
He's with me every single day,
Though others seldom notice.

He troubles many people,
No matter who they are,
Whether mom or dad or cousin,
Sibling, stranger—near or far.

The doctors aren't sure why My Sick
Chose to visit me.
His reasons are unknown to us.
He is a mystery.

Sometimes he might be scary,
There are things that he might do.
Just know that though I have My Sick
He cannot bother you.

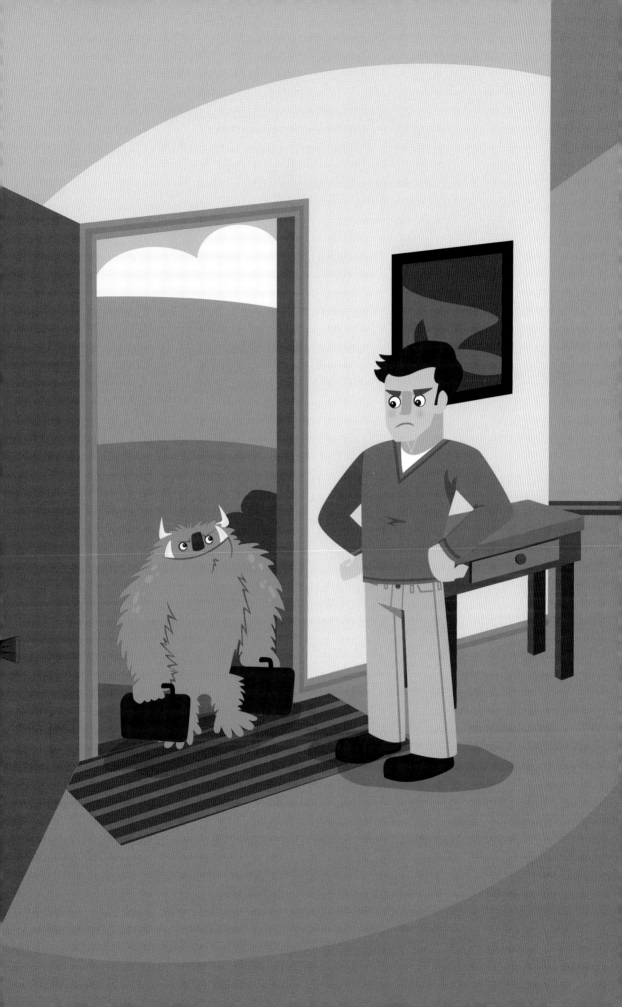

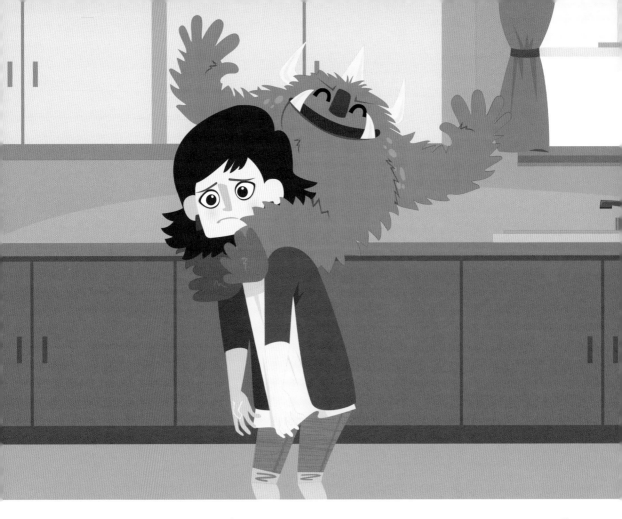

The times when My Sick wants to play
I have twice the weight to bear,
And I lose twice the energy
When I go anywhere.

And since I have this burden,
There's much less I can do.
Though I've planned many adventures,
I can only go on a few.

But this new part of my life
Has helped me find my way.
I learn what's most important
As I plan out my day.

I've learned to limit what I do
And save some time for me.
And of course for those I love:
My friends and family.

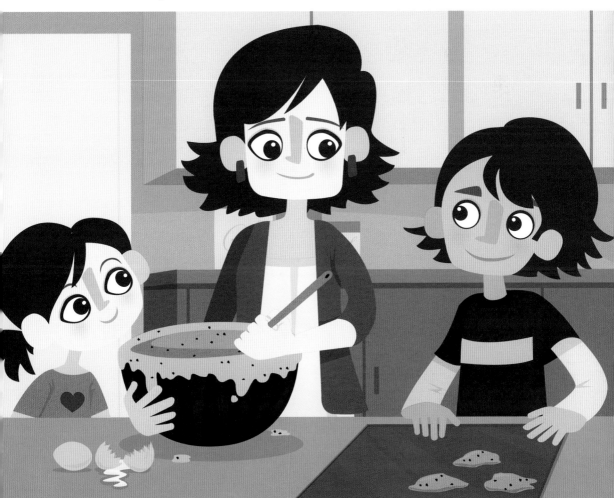

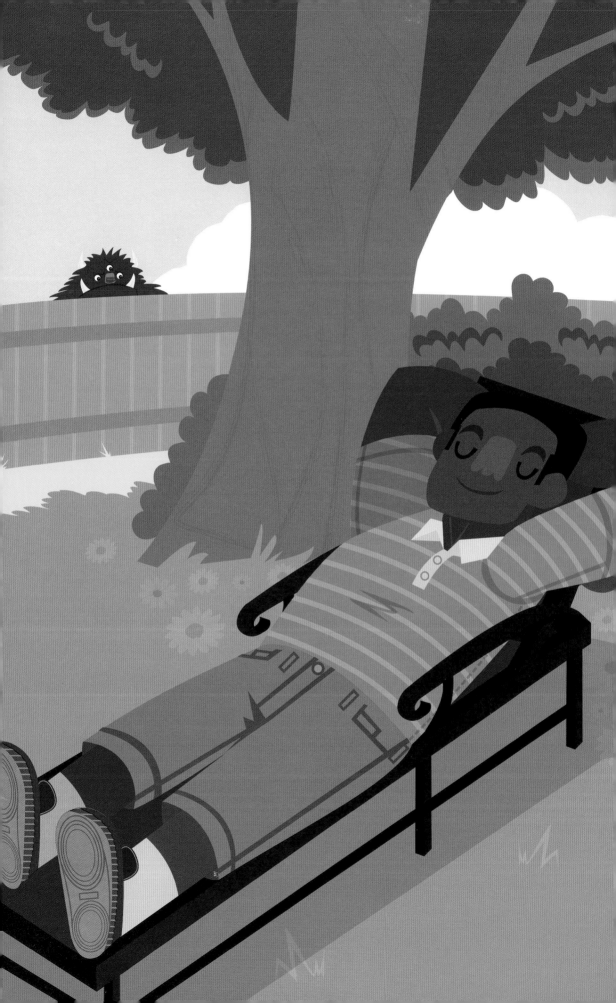

Hot days take My Sick's temper
And stretch it paper thin.
He uses all his tricks on me,
But I won't let him win.

In cool spots in the shade
Or air-conditioned homes,
I stop My Sick from getting mad,
And he leaves me alone.

Today I'm feeling pretty great.
My Sick's not by my side.
It's kind of like I've scared My Sick
And gotten him to hide.

And since My Sick is missing,
It means I'm free to play.
So as I play with you, let's hope
Tomorrow's like today.

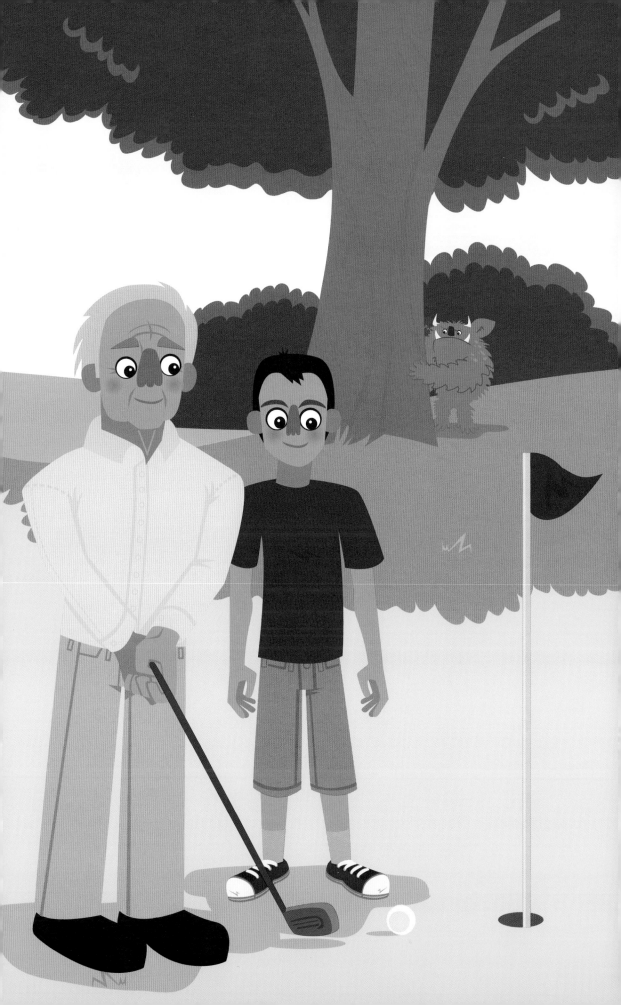

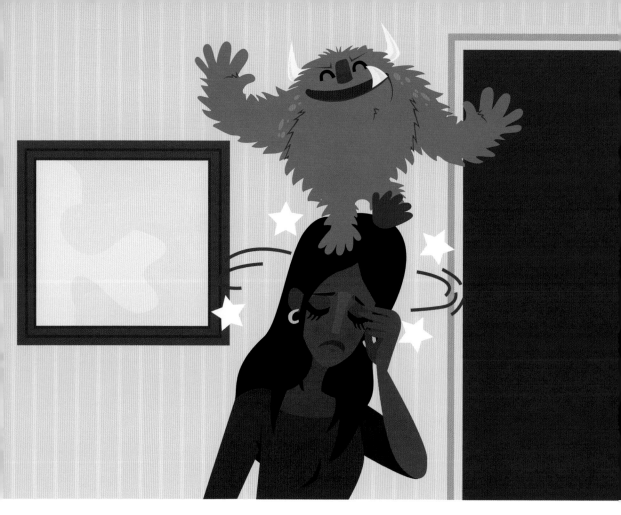

The days make me feel dizzy.
My eyes swing all around.
My Sick keeps dancing on my brain—
I need to go lay down.

At nights while resting in my bed
He pokes and tickles me.
And since he wants to keep me up,
I'll go and make some tea.

But underneath the covers
While I am counting sheep,
I stay still and quiet
And try to fall asleep.

I breathe real slow and tell My Sick,
"I know you're here today,
But now—right now—I need to rest,
It's time to go away."

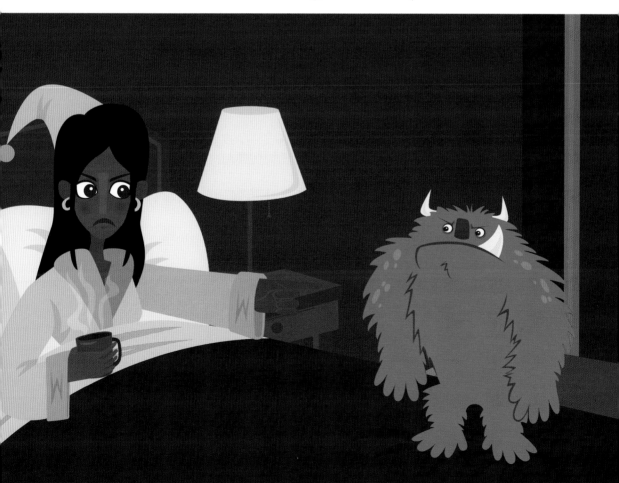

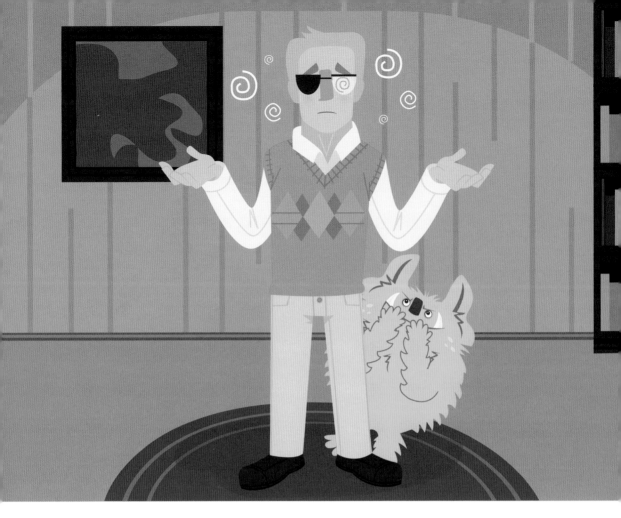

My Sick is rather devious,
He takes me by surprise.
He puts tape on my glasses
Or even steals my eyes.

And when my vision's blurry,
Or even worse—all gone.
My Sick just laughs and sneers at me
And sings his villain's song.

But just like any bully,
My Sick just wants attention.
So even when it's tough to see,
I do not pay him mention.

Instead I'll rest and close my eyes,
And picture my family.
'Cuz when he gives my vision back,
They're who I'll want to see.

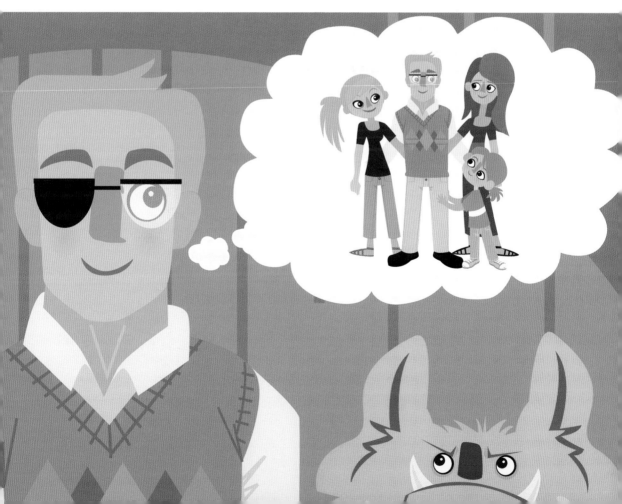

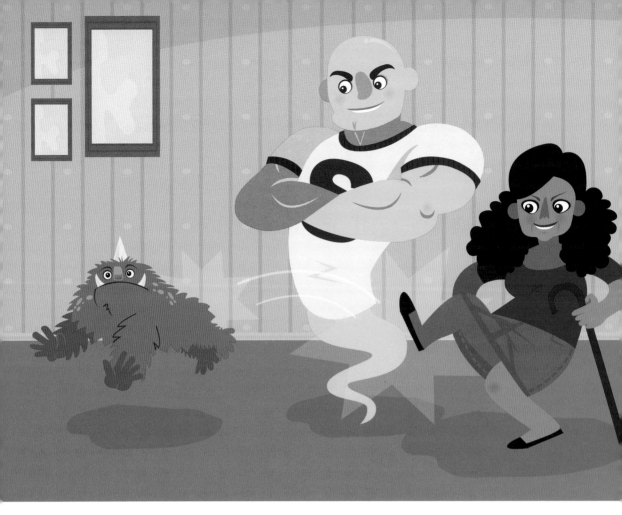

Sometimes My Sick is just too much
To handle by myself,
So my doctor gives me steroids
To help restore my health.

The steroids are quite helpful,
They help me to bounce back.
When My Sick gets out of hand,
They quiet his attack.

Though the steroids help me,
Some parts of them are bad.
Whenever I rely on them,
I may get mad or sad.

So if I ever need a hug
Or time all by myself,
Please be there to help me out
As I take back my health.

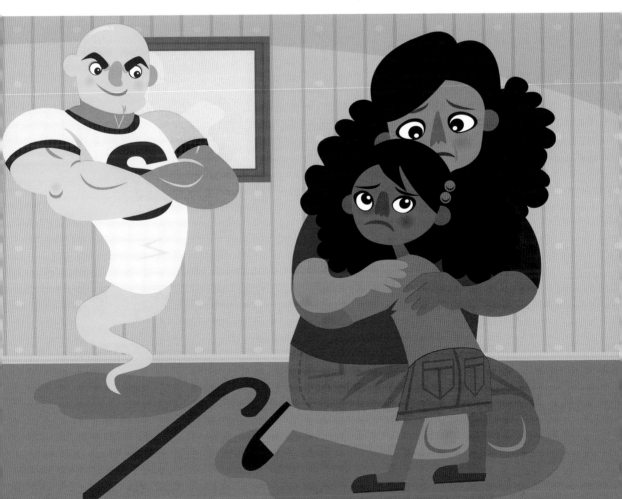

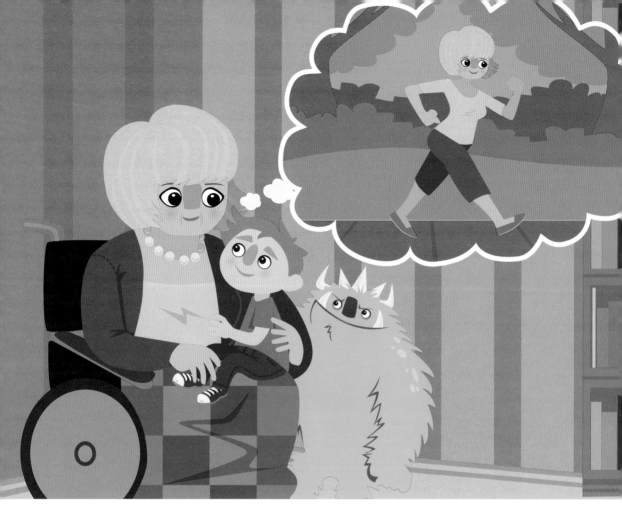

Though once I walked with quickness,
Now my pace has slowed.
At first My Sick gave me a cane
To lead me as I go.

Then My Sick took back the cane
And forced me to a chair.
He made me weak in all my limbs
So he could keep me there.

But though My Sick may take my legs,
He cannot take my smile.
For I will watch you laugh and play
And love you all the while.

And with the strength that I still have,
There's plenty we can do.
Like read or sing or play fun games,
The choice is up to you.

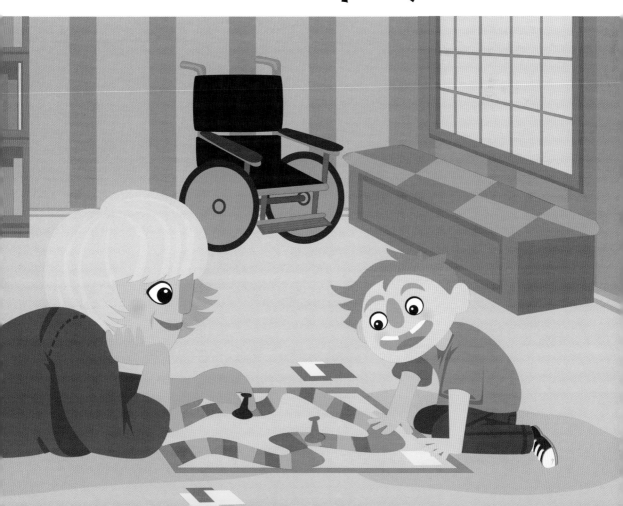

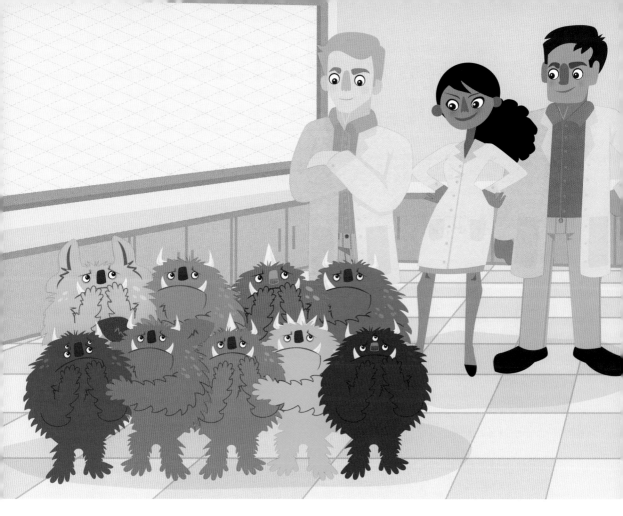

No matter what My Sick might do,
No matter his attack.
I find strength in scientists.
I know they've got my back.

The scientists are heroes.
Their mission's very clear:
Find better ways to fight My Sick
And work to find a cure.

So though he tries to beat me
There will never be even sides.
I have with me all those I love—
No wonder My Sick hides.

And when he's off in hiding,
We'll all work together.
Working towards that awesome day
When My Sick's gone forever.

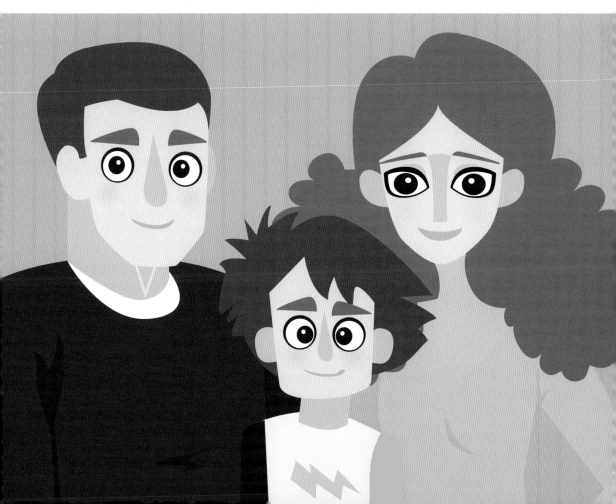

There is strength in many people
No matter who they are.
Whether mom or dad or cousin
Sibling, stranger—near or far.

This here is My Sick—
Multiple Sclerosis.
He's with me every single day,
Though often I don't notice.

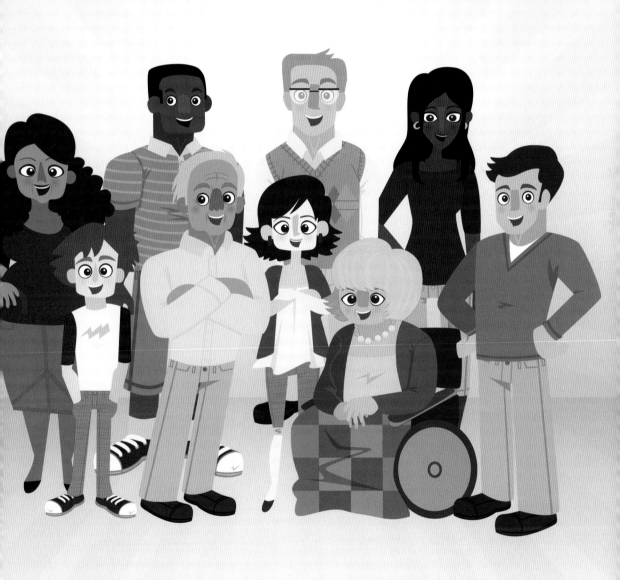

THE END

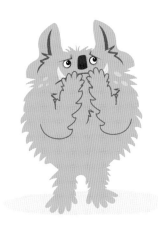

About the Founders

MS Children's Book is more than just a book, it's a company!
Founded by six University of Washington students, MS Children's Book sponsors MS events such as the annual Walk MS, organizes community fundraisers, restaurant and book events, partners with schools for events, and is even creating a cycling team to raise money and awareness for MS. We donate 100% of our profits to the organizations listed on the following page. But we don't just sell books, we donate them. In fact, if you didn't purchase the book you are reading, chances are it was donated to you by us, or another kind soul who purchased it to be donated to you. In the future, we hope to host a camp for kids who either have MS, or a loved one who does. Who knows, maybe we'll even write another book! To learn more, visit www.mschildrensbook.com or find us on Facebook at www.facebook.com/mschildrensbook

William Khazaal
William Khazaal is CEO of MS Children's Book. Khazaal worked closely with the author and the illustration team providing both vision and editorial consulting. He plays an active role in all aspects of the company. For years, he has worked in the field of finance and marketing in a management capacity, and has founded companies of his own prior to MS Children's Book. He is a graduate of University of Washington, Foster School of Business with degrees in Entrepreneurship and Marketing. Khazaal lives in Seattle with his wife Megan and their two sons, Gabriel and Blakely. In 2009, Khazaal was diagnosed with MS, and it was Gabriel who coined the term "My Sick".

Molly Massena
Molly Massena was raised in Spokane, WA where she obtained her Minor in German before moving to Seattle. At age 22 Massena received her Undergraduate in Finance and Entrepreneurship from the University Of Washington Foster School Of Business. She has 5 years of experience working with small to medium size corporations such as PEARL Microfinance, Sigfont.com, AIESEC, and now MS Children's Book. In her free time she volunteers for organizations that perk her interests, spends time doing outdoor sports, and continues to travel the world adding to her current list of 30 countries. Massena works with MS Children's Book because she truly believes in the impact that a children's book can have on the lives of those touched by MS.

Eugene Kim
Eugene Kim, our social media champion, lives to "get out there, meet new people, and make the invisible visible." Inspired by Khazaal's story, it is Kim's mission to reach as many people as possible by utilizing his work experience at Keiretsu Forum and his network at Sigma Beta Rho Fraternity, Inc. He is a graduate of the Foster Business School with degrees in Entrepreneurship and Information Systems.

Zachary Raasch
Zachary Raasch is the company's Chief Creative Officer. Raasch is a 22-year old graduate of the University of Washington, where he studied both Business and Creative Writing. He has studied the art of poetry under May Swenson award-winner Jason Whitmarsh, as well as MacArthur & Guggenheim fellow Richard Kenney. Previously, Raasch has done not-for-profit work with the CISCO Networking Academy & the Rotary Foundation, setting up and connecting computers to the internet throughout the northern parts of Slovakia.

Adam Greenberg
Adam Greenberg, the company's CFO, grew up in San Francisco. His passion for entrepreneurship began at an early age with ventures in the photography and automotive industries. He has served as a volunteer for Challenger Little League, The Janet Pomeroy Center, and Habitat for Humanity. Greenberg has studied in South Africa and Ireland, and is currently studying at the University of Washington, Foster School of Business, majoring in Finance and Entrepreneurship.

Dmitry Muzechuk
Dmitry Muzechuk was born in Ukraine and raised in both Seattle and Alaska. He is a junior at the University of Washington majoring in Entrepreneurship, Sales, and Marketing at the Foster School of Business. He grew up engulfed in his father's automotive business and now has a passion for building companies. He currently has plans for start-ups in the auto parts industry as well as real estate. Muzechuk has been fighting type-1 diabetes since he was 17 and believes in the powerful impact that this book can have on the MS community, and the proceeds can have towards finding a cure.

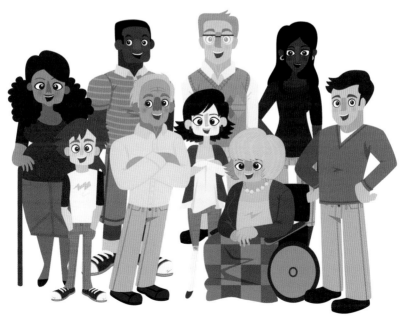

About Multiple Sclerosis

Today, there are over 2.5 million people afflicted by multiple sclerosis (MS), and every hour of every day, someone receives this life-changing diagnosis.

MS is a neurological disorder where one's own immune system attacks ones central nervous system, the part of the body that controls everything one does. For whatever reason, in MS, the immune system mistakes the insulation surrounding the nerve fibers in the brain and spinal cord for a foreign invader.

Symptoms range from dizziness and fatigue, to blindness and paralysis. The disease is usually progressive, and sometimes fatal. There is no cure for MS.

By purchasing this book, you are bringing us one step closer to finding that cure and ending MS once and for all. And for that, we thank you from the bottom of our hearts.

If you did not buy this book, then it was purchased for you by what you may call a Good Samaritan, or guardian angel – someone who selflessly donated money so you could have a copy of your very own. Whoever that person may be, we are grateful for their generosity and support.

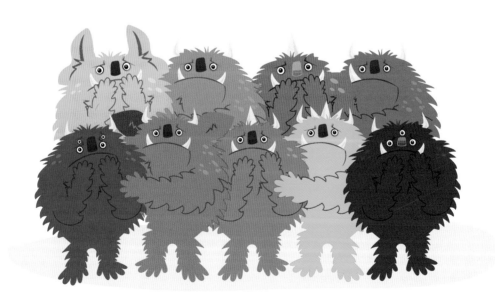

Organizations we Support

100% of MS Children's Book's profits will be donated to the following organizations

Mission:
We are committed to improving the lives of children and adolescents with multiple sclerosis by providing a center of excellence for comprehensive treatment and by advancing a research program that will benefit all individuals with MS .

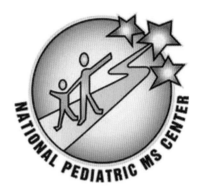

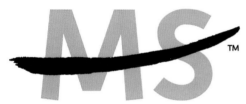

National Multiple Sclerosis Society

Mission:
We mobilize people and resources to drive research for a cure and to address the challenges of everyone affected by MS.

Mission:
CCSVI Alliance promotes education and research about CCSVI and its relationship to Multiple Sclerosis (MS) by providing objective information to the MS community, supporting medical investigations of CCSVI, and fostering collaboration among patients, advocates, and professionals.

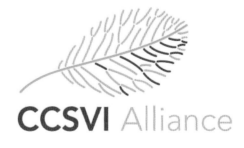